NCCN Guidelines for Patients®

The essential guide for people facing cancer.

Based on care recommendations from leading cancer experts.

Explains high-quality cancer care provided at state-of-the-art cancer centers.

Reviewed and revised every year.

Did you know that top cancer centers across the United States work together to improve cancer care? This alliance of leading cancer centers is called the National Comprehensive Cancer Network® (NCCN®).

Because cancer care is always evolving, NCCN develops and frequently updates evidence-based cancer care recommendations used by health care providers worldwide. These recommendations are known as the NCCN Clinical Practice Guidelines in Oncology (NCCN Guidelines®).

The NCCN Guidelines for Patients plainly explain these expert recommendations, so you can talk with your care team about the best care for you.

These NCCN Guidelines for Patients are based on the NCCN Guidelines® for Myeloproliferative Neoplasms, Version 1.2026 — January 22, 2026.

View the NCCN Guidelines for Patients free online: NCCN.org/patientguidelines

Find an NCCN Cancer Center near you: NCCN.org/cancercenters

Learn how the NCCN Guidelines for Patients are developed: NCCN.org/patient-guidelines-process

Connect with us

@NCCNorg @NCCNVideo NCCN @NCCNorg

Supporters

NCCN Guidelines for Patients are supported by funding from the NCCN Foundation®

NCCN Foundation gratefully acknowledges the following corporate supporters for helping to make available these NCCN Guidelines for Patients: Incyte Corporation, Novartis Pharmaceuticals Corporation, PharmaEssentia, Sobi, and Takeda Oncology.

NCCN independently adapts, updates, and hosts the NCCN Guidelines for Patients. Our corporate supporters do not participate in the development of the NCCN Guidelines for Patients and are not responsible for the content and recommendations contained therein.

Additional support is provided by

MPN Research Foundation is dedicated to funding and advancing original research in pursuit of new treatments — and eventually a cure — for essential thrombocythemia (ET), polycythemia vera (PV), and myelofibrosis (MF), blood cancers known collectively as myeloproliferative neoplasms (MPN). Founded in 1999, MPN Research Foundation was the first organization in the MPN space, and is the primary, global organization focused on advancing research. Its collaborative, patient-centered approach brings experts together, elevates the patient voice, and propels scientific progress in these complex diseases. To further this patient-centered research mission, MPN Research Foundation helps the MPN community stay informed by sharing curated updates on scientific progress, drug development, the clinical landscape, educational resources, and opportunities to engage with the broader MPN community.

To make a gift, visit
NCCNFoundation.org/Donate

To learn more, visit online
NCCN.org/patientguidelines
or email
PatientGuidelines@NCCN.org

Contents

NCCN Foundation seeks to support the millions of patients and their families affected by a cancer diagnosis by funding and distributing NCCN Guidelines for Patients. NCCN Foundation is also committed to advancing cancer treatment by funding the nation's promising doctors at the center of innovation in cancer research. For more details and the full library of patient and caregiver resources, visit NCCN.org/patients.

National Comprehensive Cancer Network (NCCN) and NCCN Foundation
3025 Chemical Road, Suite 100, Plymouth Meeting, PA 19462 USA

1 About MPNs

Myeloproliferative neoplasms (MPNs) are a type of blood cancer. Their impact on quality of life greatly varies among people. For some, MPNs cause life-changing symptoms. But, because these cancers grow so slowly, many people with MPNs can have long lives.

What are MPNs?

Myeloproliferative neoplasms (MPNs) are a group of rare blood cancers (also known as chronic leukemias). What exactly does the name mean?

- The first part of the first word—**myelo**—refers to bone marrow. Almost all bones have a soft center, called marrow, where most blood cells are formed.
- The second part of the first word—**proliferative**—refers to the growth of cells.
- A **neoplasm** is an abnormal growth of cells.

Put together, the name **myeloproliferative neoplasm** means cancer of the blood cells in bone marrow. There are many types of blood cells, so there are many types of blood cancer.

Common symptoms of MPNs

MPN symptoms can be very different among individuals. Some symptoms, called constitutional symptoms, can be present alone or together. They may include:

- Fatigue (feeling extremely tired)
- Bone pain
- Severe itching
- Headaches
- Night sweats
- Unintentional weight loss
- Pain in the upper left side of the abdomen due to an enlarged spleen
- Feeling full quickly upon eating

“

MPNs are classified as a blood cancer, but it is a cancer with a very small c! It is easy to become fearful and obsessed when first diagnosed (I know I was!), but MPNs are for most people highly treatable. Find a doctor that is an MPN specialist and join reputable online MPN patient forums. It makes all the difference."

How are MPNs treated?

In people with MPNs, the symptoms are treated before the cancer is addressed. This means that pain or blood clots are treated with pain relievers or anticoagulant medications before radiation or chemotherapy is considered.

No one MPN treatment is best for everyone. The best treatment is the treatment that's right for you. Your treatment plan should follow best practices—cancer care based on science and expert consensus.

Treatment may not be needed

MPNs are chronic cancers. These cancers can be stable for several years and typically progress slowly. Treatment may not be needed right away or ever, but MPNs are not typically cured.

People with MPNs often live for many years with proper treatment. But for some, the cancer worsens quickly. The course of the cancer depends on the MPN type, cancer features, and your age and health.

What are the classic MPNs?

There are many types of MPNs, but this guide is about the most common (or classic) types.

- **Primary myelofibrosis (PMF)** causes an excess of megakaryocytes (cells that create platelets) that triggers a buildup of scarring in bone marrow.
- **Polycythemia vera (PV)** causes an excess of red blood cells.
- **Essential thrombocythemia (ET)** causes an excess of platelets.

More information on the classic types of MPN is in *Chapter 2: Testing for MPNs*.

Chronic myeloid leukemia (CML) is an MPN with too many granulocytes, a type of white blood cell. Some people call it a classic MPN, but it's often discussed by itself. Its treatment is based on a cancer marker that the other classic MPNs do not have.

More information on CML is available at NCCN.org/patientguidelines and on the NCCN Patient Guides for Cancer app.

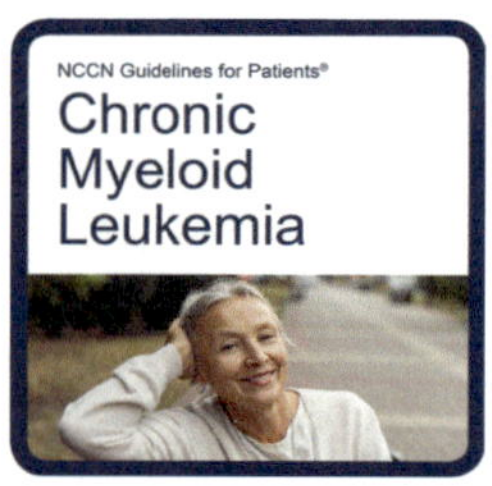

How can I get the best care?

Advocate for yourself. You have an important role to play in your care. Many people feel more satisfied when they actively take part in planning their cancer care.

The NCCN Guidelines for Patients will help you play a larger role in your care. Discuss the recommendations in this guide with your care team. Ask questions about your options and share your goals and concerns.

Don't know what to ask? You're not alone. That's why we include suggested questions to ask at the end of chapters.

Keep reading to find the best care for you.

How this guide can help you

Making decisions about cancer care is stressful. There's a lot to learn, and you don't know what the future holds.

Use this guide to get the information and support you need.

Patients, doctors, and other health care professionals trust the NCCN Guidelines for Patients. This guide uses clear, everyday language to explain current cancer care recommendations made by respected experts in the field. Their recommendations are based on the latest research and practices at leading cancer centers.

Your health is unique to you, so your cancer care should be, too. As you read this guide, you'll learn which treatments are likely to provide the best results for you. And you'll be better prepared to talk with your care team.

2
Testing for MPNs

Several tests are needed if your health care provider suspects a myeloproliferative neoplasm (MPN). These tests are described in this chapter.

Testing does not differ much among the types of myeloproliferative neoplasm (MPN). Each type—primary myelofibrosis (PMF), polycythemia vera (PV), and essential thrombocythemia (ET)—requires blood work. Tests on a bone marrow sample are also very common. See **Guide 1** for a list of tests used to diagnose and plan treatment of MPNs.

Ask for copies of your test results, and take notes as your health care provider explains the reports.

Don't let your nerves stop you from asking questions. MPNs are complex and can be hard to understand.

Bringing someone with you to your appointments can be helpful. Keep your reports and other paperwork handy and organized in a file (such as a binder) for when you need them again.

Guide 1
Tests for myeloproliferative neoplasms

Health history and exam	• Medical history, including transfusions and medicines • Physical exam • Symptom scale
Blood tests	• Complete blood count (CBC) with differential • Blood smear • Comprehensive metabolic panel, liver function tests, lactate dehydrogenase (LDH), uric acid • Erythropoietin (EPO) and iron • Human leukocyte antigen and coagulation tests are sometimes needed
Bone marrow tests	• Bone marrow biopsy and aspiration • Study of bone marrow using special stains and a microscope
Biomarker tests	• Fluorescence in situ hybridization (FISH) or multi-plex RT-PCR for *BCR-ABL1* • Molecular tests or multi-gene next-generation sequencing (NGS) for *JAK2*, *CALR*, and *MPL* mutations • Cytogenetics using karyotype with or without FISH

Health history

Expect your health care provider to review your health in detail. This is known as taking a medical history. Your health care provider will want to know a lot about your past and current health. You will likely be asked about:

- Illnesses and diseases
- Prescribed and over-the-counter medicines and supplements, surgeries, and blood transfusions
- Lifestyle choices, including your diet, how active you are, and whether you smoke or drink alcohol
- Symptoms and complications of MPNs, such as fatigue, weight loss, headache, bone pain, abdominal pain, and itching or tingling

MPNs rarely run in families. It's uncommon to be born with an abnormal gene that causes an MPN. Most people acquire changes in genes after birth that may lead to an MPN.

Some other types of cancer and health conditions do run in families. Be prepared to discuss the health problems of your close blood relatives. These include your siblings, parents, and grandparents.

Physical exam

Your health care provider should perform a thorough physical exam of your body. This exam may include:

- Checking your vital signs—blood pressure, heart rate, breathing rate, and temperature—and assessing your overall appearance
- Feeling and listening to organs, including your spleen and liver
- Assessing your level of pain, if any, when you are touched

“Much diagnosis and treatment is blood work number based and can be done virtually. Get a second opinion or third. Had I not sought out an amazing MPN expert and instead trusted my first oncologist—I am sure I would not be where I am now—healthy, good numbers, and confident in my MPN treatment journey and medical team."

Blood tests

Blood tests can measure blood cells, proteins, and chemicals in the bloodstream. They are commonly used to screen for disease and to plan treatment of blood cancers.

Some blood tests are done with a machine, while others need a pathologist to complete. A pathologist is a doctor who's an expert in tissues and cells.

For MPNs, a doctor called a hematopathologist may be part of your care team. This doctor is an expert at diagnosing cancers of the blood and immune cells.

Complete blood count with differential

A complete blood count (CBC) with differential is a very common lab test. It measures:

- The numbers of white blood cells, red blood cells, and platelets
- The percentages of red blood cells in blood (called hematocrit)
- The amount of a protein called hemoglobin in red blood cells
- The numbers of the most common types of white blood cells—basophils, neutrophils, eosinophils, monocytes, and lymphocytes

Blood smear

A pathologist will inspect a sample of your blood using a microscope. The sample is known as a blood smear. With a microscope, a pathologist can see the size and shape of blood cells. Abnormal features of blood cells can be a clue to what disease you have.

A blood smear can also show if there are immature blood cells, called blasts, in the blood. Blasts are normally found only in bone marrow, but sometimes myelofibrosis forces them into the blood circulating in your body.

Metabolic panel and liver tests

A comprehensive metabolic panel measures up to 14 types of chemicals that come from your organs. It's a screening test for many diseases. It can also show if the MPN is affecting other parts of your body, such as your bones and liver.

Liver function tests are also used to assess if the MPN is affecting your liver. These tests measure a yellow-colored fluid called bile as well as liver proteins and enzymes.

Lactate dehydrogenase and uric acid

Most cells have a protein called lactate dehydrogenase (LDH) and a chemical called uric acid. During certain phases, myelofibrosis causes many blood cells to die. Dying blood cells release LDH and uric acid. As a result, high levels of LDH and uric acid may be signs of myelofibrosis.

Erythropoietin and iron

Erythropoietin (EPO) is a hormone made by the kidneys. It helps to make red blood cells, and iron is needed to make hemoglobin in red blood cells. Hemoglobin delivers the oxygen you breathe to your body's cells and organs.

Blood tests that measure EPO and iron help diagnose PV. In PV, high red blood cell counts suppress EPO levels. Also, iron levels may be low despite high hemoglobin levels.

Other blood tests

Other blood tests are sometimes needed. People who have a treatment called an allogeneic hematopoietic cell transplant (HCT) need human leukocyte antigen testing. To learn more about allogeneic HCT, read *Chapter 4: Myelofibrosis.*

A coagulation test may be done to assess how well your blood clots. Some people are diagnosed with acquired von Willebrand syndrome (aVWS) or another blood clotting disorder based on the results of these tests.

Bone marrow tests

Bone marrow is the soft center in the middle of most bones. It's like a sponge holding liquid and cells.

A bone marrow biopsy removes a core sample of marrow. Bone marrow aspiration removes liquid and cells. Both procedures are often done at the same time on the back of the hip bone. You may receive an injected pain blocker or light sedative to relax you beforehand.

A pathologist will inspect your bone marrow using a microscope. This is known as bone marrow histology. Histology can detect abnormal numbers of bone marrow cells. It can also show how much bone marrow is scarred (fibrosis).

Removing bone marrow samples

Samples of your bone marrow might be removed and tested for diagnosis or treatment planning. A bone marrow aspiration removes a small amount of liquid bone marrow. A bone marrow biopsy removes a small piece of bone along with the marrow. These procedures are often done on the back of the hip one after the other.

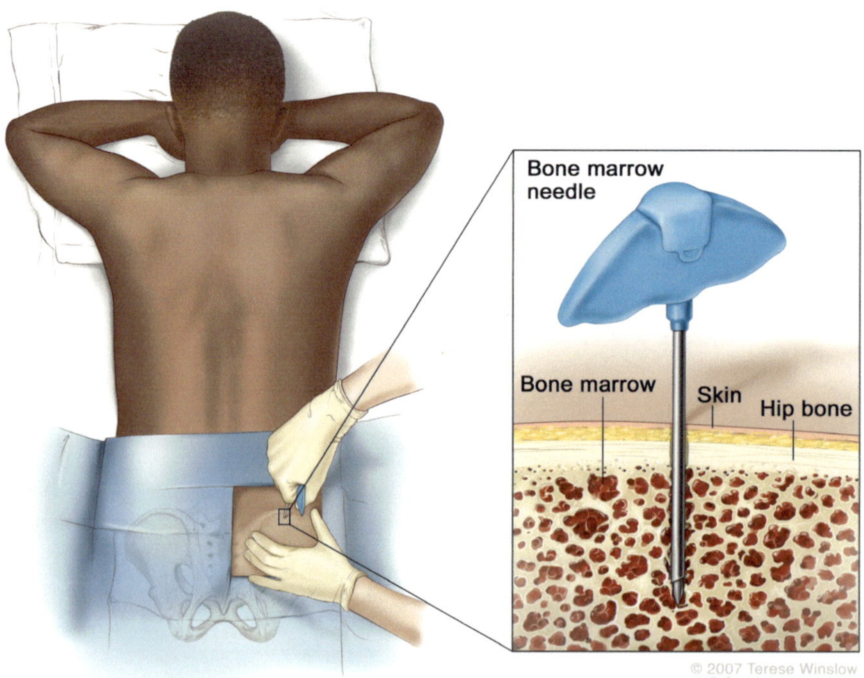

Biomarker tests

Biomarker tests look for biological clues, or markers, of cancer. Molecular tests are a type of biomarker test that looks for abnormal genes called mutations. Some people call them genetic tests. Cytogenetic tests show if there are abnormal chromosomes.

Biomarker test for CML mutation

The hallmark of chronic myeloid leukemia (CML) is the *BCR-ABL1* fusion gene. Fluorescence in situ hybridization (FISH) and multi-plex reverse transcription-polymerase chain reaction (RT-PCR) are molecular tests that detect *BCR-ABL1* in blood or bone marrow. If *BCR-ABL1* is missing, CML is ruled out.

Biomarker tests for MPN mutations

If CML is ruled out, molecular testing is used to look for markers of classic MPNs. This section describes a few of the many possible mutations tested with modern multi-gene testing.

Tests for diagnosis
One of the markers is the *JAK2* V617F mutation. If this marker is not found, the next markers to be tested are:

- *JAK2* exon 12 mutation if PV is suspected
- *CALR* and *MPL* mutations if ET or PMF is suspected
- Occasionally, all 3 of the above mutations are negative. This is called triple-negative MPN, but absence of these 3 mutations does not rule out MPN.

A newer technology called multi-gene testing can test for additional multiple genetic markers at the same time. It may be used instead of single molecular tests.

Tests for prognosis
If tests confirm you have an MPN, multi-gene testing is recommended to assess prognosis if it wasn't done before. Prognosis is a prediction of how the cancer will behave and respond to treatment.

Biomarker tests for abnormal chromosomes

Cytogenetics are useful for diagnosis and treatment planning. Results can help identify MPN subtypes, grade bone marrow fibrosis, and assess the prognosis of the cancer.

A picture of chromosomes, called a karyotype, is used for cytogenetics. A FISH test may be done to look for specific chromosome abnormalities. These tests are done on a bone marrow aspirate or blood sample.

> “I take each day at a time. Sometimes the fatigue is greater than other days. You must persevere."

Challenges to diagnosis

Diagnosing MPN can be tricky. Some of the challenges to diagnosis are:

- Signs and symptoms of MPNs can have other causes. Other causes need to be ruled out.
- Classic MPNs can have very similar test results. Early PMF may look like ET because there may be little bone marrow scarring.
- Recent bleeding can change test results and hide the correct diagnosis.
- Symptoms and test results differ among the early, middle, and late phases of an MPN. Health care providers need to know what each MPN phase looks like.

The pathologist will identify the MPN subtype when possible. Although rare, there are times when the MPN subtype is not clear. These cancers are called **MPN, not otherwise specified (NOS)**.

Always be prepared for the worst-case scenario, but maintain a positive outlook and hope for the best. Above all, never give up!"

Why am I so tired?

Symptoms caused by MPN can also be caused by other conditions. The overlap may make diagnosing MPN a challenge. Fatigue, for example, is the most common symptom of MPN. But fatigue is also caused by some medications, many diseases, and poor mental health and physical fitness.

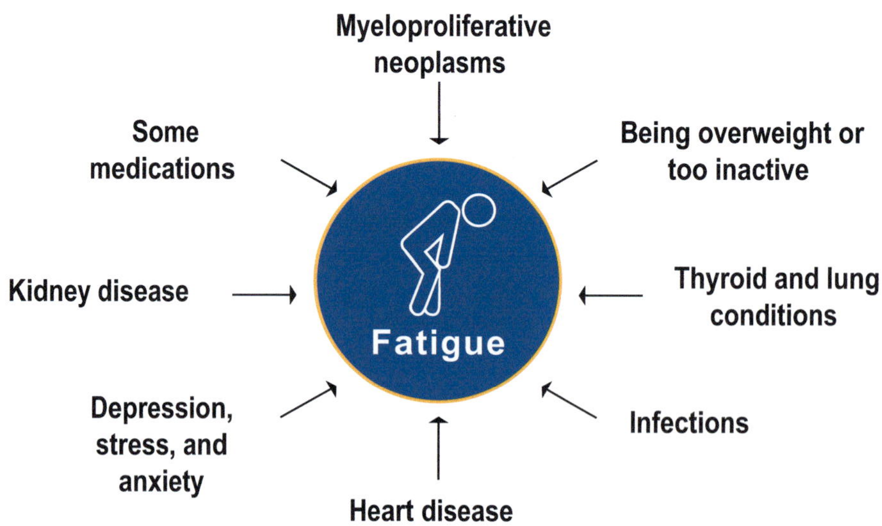

Key points

- If a myeloproliferative neoplasm (MPN) is suspected, a group of tests is needed for diagnosis. Testing does not differ much among the MPN types.
- Be ready to tell your care team about any health problems and treatments you've had in your lifetime.
- Your health care provider will examine your body for signs of disease. The exam will include touching parts of your body to see if anything feels abnormal.
- You will need to provide samples of blood, bone marrow, or both. Your blood and bone marrow will be sent to a lab to be tested for signs of MPNs and other diseases.
- Despite criteria to diagnose MPN types, diagnosis can be challenging. Most MPNs have a genetic marker. These markers include *JAK2*, *CALR*, and *MPL* mutations.

Questions to ask

- What tests will I have? What is involved if I need a biopsy?
- Do the tests have any risks?
- Do I need to do anything to prepare for testing?
- Where do I go for testing, and how long will it take?
- Should I bring someone with me to the appointments?

What's next?

Once the type of MPN is diagnosed, you may receive treatment or your doctor may say, "Let's watch and wait" to see if over time your symptoms change. In this case, you may return for a physical exam and bloodwork in 3 to 6 months. The types of treatments offered to people with MPN are covered in the next chapter.

3
Types of treatment

Myeloproliferative neoplasms (MPNs) can cause a variety of symptoms that need to be treated in a variety of ways. This chapter describes what each of these treatments do.

All treatments listed in this guide are recommended and appropriate. When helpful, NCCN experts also assign a level of preference to their recommendations for systemic therapies:

- **Preferred therapies** have the most evidence they may work better and be safer than other therapies.
- **Other recommended therapies** can provide effective results but may have less evidence, more side effects, or may not work quite as well as preferred therapies.
- **Therapies used in certain cases** work best for individuals with specific cancer features or health circumstances.

Antiplatelets

In healthy blood, platelets to stick together to form a clot and stop bleeding. However, in people with clotting disorders platelets may stick together even if there's no bleeding. Antiplatelet medications make the platelets less likely to stick together, reducing the likelihood of blood clots.

Examples of antiplatelet medications include aspirin and clopidogrel (Plavix).

Phlebotomy

Sometimes, the best treatment for myeloproliferative neoplasms (MPNs) is to simply remove the blood that's causing your symptoms. This is called phlebotomy, sometimes known as bloodletting. A member of your care team will place a needle in your arm to draw out some extra/excess blood.

If you have problems with needles, let your care team know so they can try to make you more comfortable.

There are specific treatment options to remove specific cells, such as platelets.

Plateletpheresis

Plateletpheresis is similar to an anticoagulant in that it removes platelets from the body to encourage better blood flow. However, plateletpheresis involves putting your blood into a machine that specifically filters platelets out, like a water purifier.

It uses a needle placed into your arm.

> **"The impact of MPNs can be quite wide-ranging. There is more to these conditions than the risk of thrombosis. The secondary or constitutional symptoms can be more problematic and deserve equal attention."**

Cytoreductive therapy

People who are highly likely to get blood clots may take medication that lowers blood counts, called cytoreductive therapy. This therapy is sometimes given to relieve symptoms when blood clots aren't likely.

Some cytoreductive therapies are preferred by NCCN experts. Preferred therapies have the most evidence they may work better and be safer than other therapies.

Cytoreductive therapies include hydroxyurea, peginterferon alfa-2a (Pegasys), ruxolitinib (Jakafi), and ropeginterferon alfa-2b-njft (Besremi).

Antihistamines

Antihistamines are medicines that specifically target histamines in your blood. Histamines control your body's immune response to outside allergens like pollen or dust, causing your eyes to itch and water when they encounter something they don't like.

A symptom of MPNs is a specific type of itchy skin, called pruritus, that has no other cause. Antihistamines, such as cetirizine (Zyrtec) or loratadine (Claritin), might be prescribed for you by your care team to help with itching as well as some types of bone pain.

JAK inhibitors

JAK is a cell protein that helps cells grow. It is key to blood stem cells developing into mature blood cells. JAK is overactive in people with the classic MPNs, whether or not there is a *JAK* mutation.

JAK inhibitors interfere with JAK and reduce the excess number of new blood cells being made. In turn, they reduce spleen size and core symptoms. Ruxolitinib (Jakafi), fedratinib (Inrebic), pacritinib (Vonjo), and momelotinib (Ojjaara) are JAK inhibitors.

"I found out in 2018 at my annual physical that my platelet count was elevated and that led to a diagnosis of ET with a JAK2 genetic mutation. I have no symptoms and my only treatment is two low-dose aspirin per day. I don't believe that this needs to be called blood cancer. I tell people that I have a blood disorder so it isn't so frightening."

Iron chelation

Iron chelation is when extra iron is removed from your body. Too many blood transfusions over a short period can cause a condition called iron overload. Iron overload resulting from too many transfusions is common with certain types of MPN.

Examples of iron chelation drugs are deferoxamine (Desferal), deferiprone (Ferriprox), and deferasirox (Exjade).

Hematopoietic cell transplant

An allogeneic hematopoietic cell transplant (HCT), also known as a bone marrow transplant, uses donor cells to form healthy bone marrow and blood cells in your body. It extends life and may cure some forms of MPN, particularly myelofibrosis.

An HCT is not safe for everyone. It's an intense treatment, so many people can't get it. A transplant specialist will assess if you can have a transplant. The specialist will also assess donor options.

"Do it for the little things... grandchildren, that is. Had I not undergone the stem cell transplant I wouldn't be here to enjoy them."

Clinical trials

A clinical trial is a type of medical research study. After being developed and tested in a lab, potential new ways of fighting cancer need to be studied in people.

If found to be safe and effective in a clinical trial, a drug, device, or treatment approach may be approved by the U.S. FDA.

Everyone with cancer should carefully consider all of the treatment options available for their cancer type, including standard treatments and clinical trials. Talk to your doctor about whether a clinical trial may make sense for you.

Phases

Most cancer clinical trials focus on treatment and are done in phases.

- **Phase 1** trials study the safety and side effects of an investigational drug or treatment approach.
- **Phase 2** trials study how well the drug or approach works against a specific type of cancer.
- **Phase 3** trials test the drug or approach against a standard treatment. If the results are good, it may be approved by the FDA.
- **Phase 4** trials study the safety and benefit of an FDA-approved treatment.

Who can enroll?

It depends on the clinical trial's rules, called eligibility criteria. The rules may be about age, cancer type and stage, treatment history, or general health. They ensure that participants are alike in specific ways and that the trial is as safe as possible for the participants.

Informed consent

Clinical trials are managed by a research team. This group of experts will review the study with you in detail, including its purpose and the risks and benefits of joining. All of this information is also provided in an informed consent form. Read the form carefully and ask questions before signing it. Take time to discuss it with people you trust. Keep in mind that you can leave and seek treatment outside of the clinical trial at any time.

Will I get a placebo?

Placebos (inactive versions of real medicines) are almost never used alone in cancer clinical trials. It's common to receive either a placebo with a standard treatment, or a new drug with a standard treatment. You will be informed, verbally and in writing, if a placebo is part of a clinical trial before you enroll.

Are clinical trials free?

There is no fee to enroll in a clinical trial. The study sponsor pays for research-related costs, including the study drug. But you may need to pay for other services, like transportation or childcare, due to extra appointments. During the trial, you will continue to receive standard cancer care. This care is often covered by insurance.

Finding a clinical trial

In the United States

NCCN Cancer Centers
NCCN.org/cancercenters

The National Cancer Institute (NCI)
cancer.gov/about-cancer/treatment/clinical-trials/search

Worldwide

The U.S. National Library of Medicine (NLM)
clinicaltrials.gov

Need help finding a clinical trial?

NCI's Cancer Information Service (CIS)
1.800.4.CANCER (1.800.422.6237)
cancer.gov/contact

Key points

- Cytoreductive medications lower the number of platelets in your bloodstream, reducing the likelihood of clotting.
- Preferred therapies have the most evidence they may work better and be safer than other therapies.
- JAK is a cell protein that helps cells grow. It is key to blood stem cells developing into mature blood cells. JAK is overactive in people with myeloproliferative neoplasms (MPNs), whether or not there is a *JAK* mutation.
- An allogeneic hematopoietic cell transplant (HCT), also known as a bone marrow transplant, uses donor cells to form healthy bone marrow and blood cells.
- A clinical trial is a type of medical research study. After being developed and tested in a lab, potential new ways of fighting cancer need to be studied in people.

Questions to ask

- What are my treatment options?
- What will happen if I do nothing?
- Are you suggesting options other than what NCCN recommends? If yes, why?
- How do my age, sex, overall health, and other factors affect my options?
- What if I am pregnant, or planning to become pregnant?

"You need to be your own advocate, particularly since this is a rare cancer and the significant majority of health care experts are not aware of MPNs. If I didn't observe my own blood work, push for appointments with hematologists, and not stop asking 'why,' I still would not know about my diagnosis and may not have learned until it was potentially too late."

4
Myelofibrosis

For some people, myelofibrosis is nearly invisible, with symptoms increasing very slowly, sometimes over several years. Others may experience a rapid increase in symptoms and disease progression. This chapter discusses how myelofibrosis is treated.

Types of myelofibrosis

Myelofibrosis is a blood cancer that causes scarring of the bone marrow, called fibrosis. It can occur in people with or without a history of a myeloproliferative neoplasm (MPN).

If myelofibrosis is a person's first MPN, it's called **primary myelofibrosis (PMF)**. It can also occur when polycythemia vera (PV) or essential thrombocythemia (ET) progresses. In these cases, it's called secondary myelofibrosis, or **post-PV** and **post-ET myelofibrosis**.

Myelofibrosis differs greatly among people in terms of its course, speed of progression, and symptoms.

Myelofibrosis progresses slowly in many people. It can be stable for many years. For others, the MPN is more active.

The first step of treatment planning is to assess the prognosis. Treatment is partly based on how aggressive the myelofibrosis is predicted to be.

Predicting prognosis

Prognosis is the likely course and outcome of the myelofibrosis. Experts and care teams use risk stratification scoring systems to assess prognosis.

Scoring systems

For PMF, NCCN experts prefer 2 scoring systems: the Mutation-Enhanced International Prognostic Score System (MIPSS)-70 and the MIPSS70-plus version 2.0. These systems are used to estimate risk of disease progression and/or complications, such as thrombosis (blood clots) and cardiovascular or kidney disease for people who are 70 years of age or under and require broad molecular testing.

Other scoring systems for people of any age are the Dynamic International Prognostic Scoring System (DIPSS) and the DIPSS-Plus. These systems are recommended if molecular testing is unavailable.

The risk stratification system used for post-PV and post-ET myelofibrosis is the MIPSS70-plus version 2.0, DIPSS-Plus, and Myelofibrosis Secondary to PV and ET-Prognostic Model (MYSEC-PM).

Risk is based on your medical information. Points are given for each response that conveys a risk of poor outcomes. Based on the total number of points, people are assigned a risk level.

Ask your provider what your risk level is and what system was used to calculate it. Risk levels for each system are given in **Guide 2**.

NCCN risk groups

NCCN experts divide the total points into 2 risk groups—lower and higher—to plan treatment.

In the next section, treatment for lower- and higher-risk myelofibrosis without anemia is discussed. But most people with myelofibrosis have anemia. If you do, read the section in this chapter called "Treating myelofibrosis with anemia."

Guide 2
Risk systems to assess prognosis of myelofibrosis

System	System risk levels	NCCN risk levels
MIPSS-70	• Low risk is a score of 0 or 1 • Intermediate risk is a score of 2, 3, or 4 • High risk is a score of 5 or above	• Lower risk is a score of 3 or below • Higher risk is a score of 4 or above
MIPSS70-plus version 2.0	• Very low risk is a score of 0 • Low risk is a score of 1 or 2 • Intermediate risk is a score of 3 or 4 • High risk is a score of 5, 6, 7, or 8 • Very high risk is a score of 9 or above	• Lower risk is a score of 3 or below • Higher risk is a score of 4 or above
DIPSS	• Low risk is a score of 0 • Intermediate-1 risk is a score of 1 or 2 • Intermediate-2 risk is a score of 3 or 4 • High risk is a score of 5 or 6	• Lower risk is a score of 2 or below • Higher risk is a score of 3 or above
DIPSS-Plus	• Low risk is a score of 0 • Intermediate-1 risk is a score of 1 • Intermediate-2 risk is a score of 2 or 3 • High risk is a score of 4 or 5	• Lower risk is a score of 1 or 0 • Higher risk is a score of 2 or above
MYSEC-PM	• Low risk is a score of 11 or below • Intermediate-1 risk is a score of 12 or 13 • Intermediate-2 risk is a score of 14 or 15 • High risk is a score of 16 or above	• Lower risk is a score of 13 or below • Higher risk is a score of 14 or above

Treating myelofibrosis without anemia

Planning treatment of myelofibrosis is based on various information, not just prognosis. Your symptoms will be tracked. Your health care provider will assess the size of your spleen during exams. Blood cell and blast counts will be monitored.

Based on this information, the goals of your treatment may include:

- Relieving symptoms
- Improving blood counts
- Preventing or delaying progression to advanced myelofibrosis or leukemia

Treatment options for myelofibrosis are described in the next pages and are listed in **Guide 3**.

Guide 3
Treatment for myelofibrosis without anemia

Risk level	Clinical status	Treatment options
Lower	You do not have symptoms	• Watch and wait • Clinical trial
	You do have symptoms	• Clinical trial • It's sometimes useful to receive: - Ruxolitinib - Peginterferon alfa-2a - Hydroxyurea if lowering blood counts would relieve symptoms - Pacritinib if platelets are less than 50,000 m^3 - Momelotinib
Higher	Your number of platelets falls within the **low to high** range (50,000 m3 or higher)	• Allogeneic hematopoietic cell transplant to try to cure the MPN or • Clinical trial, ruxolitinib, fedratinib, momelotinib, pacritinib
	You have a **very low** number of platelets (below 50,000 m^3)	• Allogeneic hematopoietic cell transplant to try to cure the MPN or • Clinical trial, pacritinib (preferred regimen), or momelotinib

Active surveillance

Lower-risk myelofibrosis is likely to be stable or to progress slowly. People with lower-risk myelofibrosis that isn't causing symptoms may start active surveillance. Also called observation or watch and wait, this is a period of testing to assess for changes in myelofibrosis. Treatment may be started if symptoms appear.

Cytoreductive therapy

Cytoreductive therapy is an option for lower-risk myelofibrosis that's causing symptoms. The therapies for myelofibrosis are hydroxyurea or peginterferon alfa-2a. More information on these therapies is in *Chapter 3: Types of treatment*.

JAK inhibitors

For **lower-risk myelofibrosis**, ruxolitinib has often been used to treat symptoms when needed. Pacritinib is an option when platelet numbers are very low. Momelotinib may be an option, but more research is needed among people with lower-risk myelofibrosis.

For **higher-risk myelofibrosis**, NCCN experts recommend specific JAK inhibitors based on platelet levels.

Fedratinib, ruxolitinib, and momelotinib are recommended when platelet levels are high. Studies of pacritinib in this platelet range are needed.

When platelet levels are very low, NCCN experts prefer pacritinib for treatment. Momelotinib needs to be studied more among people with very low platelet counts.

What does treatment involve?

JAK inhibitors are a pill you take at home. Your health care provider will determine which medications and dosing are right for you and adjust as needed. Don't stop taking the medicine unless your health care provider directs you to do so.

Most important, keep track of your symptoms and any side effects you may have. Report any physical or emotional changes, even if you're not sure they're related to your treatment.

Allogeneic HCT

Allogeneic hematopoietic cell transplant (HCT) is rarely used to treat lower-risk myelofibrosis but may be an option if platelets are low. It may also be used if the cancer cells have complex cytogenetics, which is when 3 or more unrelated defects in chromosomes occur in 2 or more cells.

Everyone with higher-risk myelofibrosis should receive an evaluation for an HCT, since it's the only chance for a cure. In people with PMF and high-risk mutations, such as *ASXL1*, *EZH2*, and *RAS*, the benefits may be worth the risks.

You may stay on a JAK inhibitor to reduce the size of your spleen and to improve your symptoms until you get a transplant.

Your care team will give you detailed information about allogeneic HCT and will answer all of your questions. An allogenic HCT can be grueling. There are 4 steps in the process. Here is a brief description.

1. Your blood will be tested for cell proteins called human leukocyte antigens (HLAs). A donor's HLAs must be a close match to yours for a transplant to work. Even with a near-perfect match, donor cells may attack your body. This is called graft-versus-host disease (GVHD).

2. You'll receive a treatment called conditioning to kill your bone marrow cells. It also weakens the immune system so your body does not kill the donor cells.

3. You'll receive the donor cells through a transfusion. A transfusion is a slow injection of blood products into a vein. New, healthy blood cells will form over the next 2 to 4 weeks. This is called engraftment.

4. You'll have to be extra careful to avoid germs for the first few weeks after the transplant because your infection-fighting immune system will be severely limited. You may be given antibiotics to prevent or treat infection. You may receive medicine called immunosuppressants to prevent GVHD.

More information about GVHD is available at NCCN.org/patientguidelines and on the NCCN Patient Guides for Cancer app.

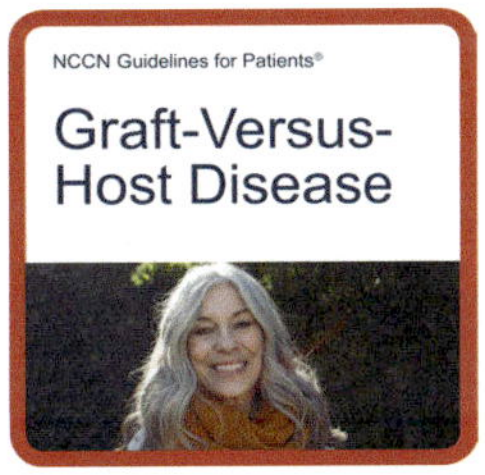

Treating myelofibrosis with anemia

Anemia is a term for low levels of hemoglobin. Most people with myelofibrosis develop anemia within 1 year after diagnosis. Anemia may cause you to feel tired and cold or look pale. These symptoms are caused by cells not getting enough oxygen.

If you have anemia, your provider will make a treatment plan based on whether you:

- Have anemia for reasons other than myelofibrosis
- Are taking a JAK inhibitor now
- Have symptoms of anemia or myelofibrosis

Depending on the causes of the anemia, your care team might prescribe supplements to replace low iron, folate, or vitamin B12 levels.

Treatment options for anemia related to myelofibrosis are discussed in **Guide 4**.

Guide 4
Treatment for myelofibrosis with anemia

Treatment for anemia	The recommended options are
When a JAK inhibitor is controlling your myelofibrosis symptoms	• Clinical trial (preferred) • Adding luspatercept-aamt, an erythropoiesis-stimulating agent, or danazol to ruxolitinib • Switching current JAK inhibitor to either momelotinib or pacritinib is sometimes useful • In addition to the options above, you may receive red blood cell transfusions if the anemia is causing symptoms
If you have uncontrolled myelofibrosis symptoms	• Clinical trial (preferred) • Momelotinib (preferred) • Pacritinib • Adding luspatercept-aamt, an erythropoiesis-stimulating agent, or danazol to ruxolitinib • In addition to the options above, you may receive red blood cell transfusions if the anemia is causing symptoms
If you don't have myelofibrosis symptoms	• Clinical trial (preferred) • Luspatercept-aamt • Erythropoiesis-stimulating agents if erythropoietin in your blood is lower than 500 mU/mL • Danazol • Momelotinib • Pacritinib • Lenalidomide, prednisone for 5q deletion • In addition to the options above, you may receive red blood cell transfusions if the anemia is causing symptoms

JAK inhibitors

JAK inhibitors reduce spleen size and core symptoms but may make anemia worse. Because of anemia, the dose of a JAK inhibitor may be reduced, or the treatment may be paused or stopped. There are other options that don't require avoiding or stopping JAK inhibitors.

- The NCCN's preferred option is momelotinib. It can improve anemia as well as myelofibrosis symptoms. More information is needed on its use among people who have anemia but no myelofibrosis symptoms.
- A second option is pacritinib. Anemia may not be as severe while pacritinib is being taken because it doesn't suppress the number of new blood cells being made. It may even increase hemoglobin.
- For people taking ruxolitinib, the third option is to keep taking it and to start anemia treatment. Luspatercept-aamt (Reblozyl), an erythropoiesis-stimulating agent, or danazol can be added to ruxolitinib to treat anemia. But these add-ons don't improve anemia for a prolonged time in many people, or they may not help at all.

Red blood cell drugs

If a JAK inhibitor isn't needed, you may receive anemia treatment that increases the number of red blood cells. These drugs include:

- Luspatercept (Reblozyl)
- Erythropoiesis-stimulating agents, such as darbepoetin alfa (Aranesp) and epoetin alfa (Epogen), if a hormone called erythropoietin is lower than 500 mU/mL in your blood
- Danazol

Red blood cell transfusions

The standard treatment for anemia that is causing symptoms is a red blood cell transfusion. Red blood cell transfusions are a common procedure. Most white blood cells are removed during a red blood cell donation to help prevent the donated blood from attacking your body.

"I am grateful for science, and for ongoing research that has turned some kinds of cancers into chronic diseases, not death sentences. I am grateful to have a good doctor and treatments that are working for me. In some ways, my cancer turned out to be lucky because it has inspired me to live in a healthier, more mindful way."

Accelerated and blast phase

Any form of MPN can progress to an accelerated or a blast phase. Over a period of 20 years, progression will occur in about 1 in 20 people with PV or ET. For PMF, it's about 3 in 20 people.

The marker of progression is a high percentage of immature blood cells, called myeloblasts (also simply called blasts), in bone marrow or the bloodstream. Blasts are usually only found in bone marrow.

Normally, the blast count in bone marrow is less than 5 percent (%). In the accelerated phase of myelofibrosis, the blast count is between 10% and 19%. In the blast phase of myelofibrosis (also called post-MPN acute myeloid leukemia [AML]), the blast count is at least 20%. AML may be diagnosed with less than 20% blasts if chromosomes have certain abnormal changes.

Lab tests

To confirm progression, lab tests on bone marrow are needed. If bone marrow can't be removed, blood samples may be used. You may know some of the lab tests used for progression because they are used for MPN diagnosis (see Chapter 2).

- Cytogenetics using karyotype with or without fluorescence in situ hybridization (FISH)
- Flow cytometry
- Multi-gene testing for mutations related to AML

Treatment planning

Right after progression is confirmed, you and your care team will discuss treatment. Treatment may include chemotherapy or chemotherapy followed by an allogeneic HCT. If a transplant is an option, you will be referred to a transplant specialist.

Low-intensity chemotherapy

When a transplant isn't an option, low-intensity chemotherapy is often used for treatment. One type of low-intensity chemotherapy is hypomethylating agents, such as azacitidine and decitabine. Learn about other low-intensity chemotherapy options for AML at NCCN.org/patientguidelines and on the NCCN Patient Guides for Cancer app.

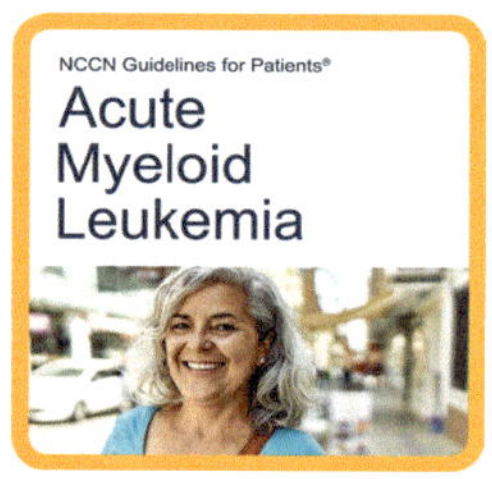

Sometimes a JAK inhibitor or a targeted therapy called venetoclax (Venclexta) is included with a hypomethylating agent. A JAK inhibitor may reduce spleen size and myelofibrosis symptoms.

Venetoclax is a pill that may help control MPN growth by targeting a protein called BCL2. But it can cause serious health problems, and you'll be monitored closely.

Induction therapy

Some people who are well enough are treated with induction therapy, which involves a combination of drugs. The goal of induction therapy is to rid the marrow of blasts. Chemotherapy used to treat AML is often used for induction.

Allogeneic HCT

If you're already taking a JAK inhibitor, it may be continued until you get a transplant.

For advanced myelofibrosis, the first step of care is to receive induction therapy before a transplant. Transplants are more successful when induction therapy has good results. Instead of induction, some people take a hypomethylating agent with or without a JAK inhibitor.

There are several steps to receiving an allogeneic HCT. These steps were described earlier in the section of this chapter called "Treating myelofibrosis without anemia."

Myelofibrosis checkups

After starting treatment, you'll need to meet with your care team often. NCCN experts advise people with lower-risk myelofibrosis under observation to have visits every 3 to 6 months. You may need visits more often if you're receiving active treatment, such as JAK inhibitors, or if you're participating in a clinical trial.

Visits with your care team

During visits, you'll be asked about new or worsening symptoms. You may be given a symptom survey called the MPN-10 to complete. For information on treating symptoms, read *Chapter 6: Supportive care*.

Your health care provider will perform a physical exam of your body. They will check the size of your spleen and liver.

You will also have blood work. Your health care provider will monitor your blood counts and other blood values. You may undergo bone marrow biopsy and aspiration if symptoms worsen or there are signs of possible progression.

Come prepared with notes about any new or changing symptoms. Bring questions you have gathered since your last visit, and consider bringing a family member or friend who can take notes and ask additional questions you may not remember to ask.

Treatment response

In research, there are standards for assessing the results of medicines. Know that your treatment may be working but may not match these standards. Your health care provider will assess treatment results mostly based on whether your symptoms are improving.

Changing treatment

Your treatment will likely not change if symptoms improve and your blood counts are acceptable. Reasons to change treatment include little to no symptom relief or worsening symptoms. Also, worsening blood counts or signs of progression may also be reasons to change treatment.

Treatment decisions may be guided by molecular testing. Testing may find new mutations since the last testing was done. Multi-gene tests on biopsy samples can detect higher-risk mutations, such as *ASXL1*, *EZH2*, and *RAS*. These mutations suggest that the myelofibrosis is likely to progress, and a transplant evaluation may be needed.

If myelofibrosis worsens but doesn't progress to leukemia, the next treatment is based on the current risk level and prior treatment. New anemia may be treated with medications that improve blood counts.

“Getting the news and diagnosis of ET with the JAK2+ mutation, wasn't going to be the end of my story. In fact, it has been the best part of my story. It has been the most challenging, yet praising God in the worst and best times, marrying my husband, preparing for a family via IVF and a surrogate, meeting new people through this diagnosis, and fighting to one day find a cure. I'm so proud of myself!"

Key points

- Myelofibrosis is a blood cancer that results in scarring of the bone marrow (fibrosis). How quickly it worsens differs greatly among people.
- The first step of treatment planning is to assess the prognosis using a risk stratification system. NCCN recommendations for treatment are based on 2 risk levels—lower and higher.
- If you have lower-risk myelofibrosis that isn't causing symptoms and don't have anemia, watch and wait is an option. Symptoms and higher-risk myelofibrosis are often treated with a JAK inhibitor. Some people are healthy enough to get an allogeneic hematopoietic cell transplant (HCT).
- If you have anemia, treatment may include a JAK inhibitor, a medication that increases red blood cell counts, or both. Standard treatment of anemia that's causing symptoms is a red blood cell transfusion.
- Advanced phases of MPN are often treated with chemotherapy, which can vary in intensity. Some people may receive an allogeneic HCT after chemotherapy.
- NCCN experts recommend clinical trials for people with MPNs. A clinical trial tests new ways of stopping cancer or reducing symptoms in people. Ask your care team if there are clinical trials that are a good fit for you.
- You will meet with your care team often after diagnosis. During visits, the status of the cancer will be checked as well as how you feel. Come prepared with notes about any new or changing symptoms. Bring questions you have gathered since your last visit, and consider bringing a family member or friend who can take notes and ask additional questions you may not remember to ask.

Questions to ask

- How do I find a myelofibrosis specialist?
- What are the goals of treatment?
- What are my chances that the myelofibrosis will become leukemia?
- What symptoms and signs would tell me that the myelofibrosis may be changing?

5 Clotting in PV and ET

In polycythemia vera (PV) and essential thrombocythemia (ET), preventing blood clots is a key part of treatment. Left unchecked, blood clots are the leading cause of death. This chapter explains how to prevent blood clots.

Polycythemia vera (PV) is a form of myeloproliferative neoplasm (MPN) that causes the bone marrow to create lots of red blood cells. Essential thrombocythemia (ET) is a form of MPN that causes the bone marrow to produce lots of platelets.

As a result, people with PV or ET are more likely to have blood clots. Unintentional blood clots can be life-threatening, and it's important to prevent them as much as possible. Learn more below.

What is a blood clot?

A blood clot is a gel-like clump of blood. Normally, blood clots develop to stop bleeding and then dissolve when the bleeding is over.

But sometimes a blood clot can form inside of a blood vessel when there is no bleeding. This type of clot is called a thrombus (or thrombi if there's more than one). A thrombus that breaks free from the vessel wall and travels in the bloodstream is called an embolus.

For our purposes, we'll refer to thrombi (or thrombosis) as blood clots for the remainder of this chapter.

People with PV and ET are prone to blood clots. Both of these disorders slow down blood flow because of the increase in blood cells, and the extra blood cells stick together. Slow-moving, sticky blood cells increase the risk of blood clots.

Blood clots are the most frequent, sometimes life-threatening, complication of PV and ET. As blood clots worsen, they can block enough blood flow (thrombosis) to cause symptoms and pain. Blocked blood flow can cause organ damage or failure, including heart attack or a stroke.

Preventive care reduces the chance of getting blood clots. With prevention, many people with PV or ET live for many years without complications.

Calculating clot risk

The risk of blood clots is not the same for everyone living with an MPN. Your health care provider will assess your risk and plan treatment based on your risk level. This process is called risk stratification.

People with PV are stratified into 1 of 2 groups—low or high risk. Risk is based on age and history of blood clots.

For ET, a tool called the International Prognostic Score of Thrombosis (IPSET) is used for risk stratification. People are assigned to very low, low, intermediate, or high risk based on age, prior blood clots, and whether they have a *JAK2* mutation.

Preventing blood clots

The plan to prevent clots differs among people. Your plan will be based on what MPN type you have, your risk of clots, and if you have symptoms of an MPN. Options for initial preventive care based on risk level are listed in **Guide 5** for PV and **Guide 6** for ET and are described next.

Managing cardiovascular risk factors

Your cardiovascular system consists of your heart, blood vessels, and blood. Cardiovascular risk is factors that will likely damage this system. Having a cardiovascular risk factor may increase your chance of getting a blood clot.

Your health care provider will assess for and help you manage cardiovascular risks that can be changed, like:

- Smoking
- Having overweight or obesity
- Getting too little exercise
- Having high blood pressure (hypertension)
- Having high blood sugar (diabetes)

Aspirin

Taking a baby aspirin every day reduces the risk of blood clots. It prevents clots by making platelets less sticky.

NCCN experts recommend taking 80 to 100 milligrams of aspirin every day for most people with PV or ET. If you're still experiencing symptoms, you can take aspirin twice a day.

Guide 5
Initial preventive care for blood clots related to polycythemia vera

Risk level of blood clots	Prevention options
Low You are under 60 years of age and have never had a blood clot.	• Management of cardiovascular risk factors • Aspirin • Phlebotomy
High You are 60 years of age or over, or you have had a blood clot.	• Management of cardiovascular risk factors • Aspirin • Phlebotomy • Cytoreductive therapy to reduce blood counts: - Hydroxyurea (preferred) - Ropeginterferon alfa-2b-njft (preferred) - Peginterferon alfa-2a - Ruxolitinib is sometimes useful

Aspirin prevents blood clots in both low- and high-risk PV. It also works well among people with ET, but not everyone with ET needs it.

Aspirin can cause more harm than good in people with very low-risk ET, especially those with acquired von Willebrand syndrome (aVWS). People with aVWS are likely to have bleeding because their blood doesn't clot as it should.

Bleeding is a side effect of aspirin for some people. Higher doses should usually be avoided because they can increase the chance of bleeding in your bowels, cause ulcers, and increase bruising.

Your blood counts may need to be lowered before you start aspirin. High blood counts increase the risk of bleeding.

Guide 6
Initial preventive care for blood clots related to essential thrombocythemia

<table>
<tr><th>Risk level of blood clots</th><th>Prevention options</th></tr>
<tr><td>Very low
You are 60 years of age or under, never had a blood clot, and do not have a JAK2 mutation.</td><td>• Management of cardiovascular risk factors
• Aspirin if you have microvascular symptoms</td></tr>
<tr><td>Low
You are 60 years of age or under, never had a blood clot, and have a JAK2 mutation.</td><td rowspan="2">• Management of cardiovascular risk factors
• Aspirin</td></tr>
<tr><td>Intermediate
You are 61 years of age or over, never had a blood clot, and do not have a JAK2 mutation.</td></tr>
<tr><td>High
You are 61 years of age or over, have had a blood clot, and have a JAK2 mutation.</td><td>• Management of cardiovascular risk factors
• Aspirin
• Cytoreductive therapy to reduce blood counts:
- Hydroxyurea (preferred)
- Peginterferon alfa-2a
- Anagrelide</td></tr>
</table>

Phlebotomy

Phlebotomy works by removing the iron-carrying red blood cells from the blood. With less iron in the body, bone marrow makes fewer red blood cells.

Blood clots aren't as likely if the bloodstream is less congested with red blood cells. After phlebotomy, you may also get quick relief from MPN symptoms—headaches, itchiness, and blurred vision.

Your health care provider will assess how often you need phlebotomy. Some people need it every other week. If your hematocrit is high, you may need it once or twice a week. Once the hematocrit and MPN symptoms are under control, the time between phlebotomies can be lengthened.

Hematocrit is a measure of red blood cells compared to the total amount of blood. Although aspirin works well for PV, the main way to prevent blood clots is to reduce hematocrit.

At diagnosis, hematocrit is often above 55 percent (%). Hematocrit should be below 45% for most people. Some people need a target below 42%.

Phlebotomy is the key strategy to reducing hematocrit. It's a procedure that removes a small amount of blood with a needle. You can think of it as the reverse of blood donation.

If you're receiving phlebotomy, don't take iron supplements unless they're prescribed by your care team.

Cytoreductive therapy

People who are highly likely to get blood clots may take medication that lowers blood counts. These cytoreductive therapies are also sometimes given to relieve symptoms when blood clots aren't likely.

Some cytoreductive therapies are preferred by NCCN experts. Preferred therapies have the most evidence they may work better and be safer than other therapies.

Anagrelide

Anagrelide (Agrylin), a capsule taken twice a day, is an antiplatelet medicine for high-risk ET. It lowers the number of platelets your body makes. It may cause headaches, digestive problems, anemia, and heart palpitations.

Hydroxyurea

Hydroxyurea (Hydrea) has been a standard cytoreductive therapy for a long time. It's a preferred initial treatment in high-risk PV and ET, though it's not well tolerated by some people. For others, it lowers blood counts and prevents blood clots for years.

Hydroxyurea works by stopping new cells from being made. It's a capsule, so you can take it at home. It's given in low doses, so many people can tolerate its side effects.

Hydroxyurea can cause below-normal blood counts, fatigue, skin changes, diarrhea, constipation, and skin cancer.

Interferon alfa

Interferon alfa naturally exists in your body and helps fight infections. It can also be created in the lab as a treatment. Interferon curbs the making of blood cells in bone marrow.

The 2 interferons used to treat MPNs are:

- Pegylated interferon, usually called peginterferon (Pegasys). This is a treatment option for high-risk PV and ET. It's sometimes given to people who are younger, are pregnant, or wish to delay taking similar medicines like hydroxyurea.
- Ropeginterferon alfa-2b-njft (Besremi). This is a preferred treatment for people with high-risk PV.

You can take interferon at home. It's injected under the skin every 2 weeks. Over time, it may be needed less often.

Interferon can cause flu-like illness, joint pain, fatigue, itching, throat swelling, musculoskeletal pain, and depression. However, an experienced MPN specialist will prescribe a lower dose than is given for other cancers, and therefore little or no side effects may be experienced.

Ruxolitinib
Ruxolitinib is sometimes useful for high-risk PV. It's a medicine called a JAK inhibitor. Read more about ruxolitinib in *Chapter 4: Myelofibrosis*.

Clot prevention during pregnancy

Consider meeting with an obstetrician who's an expert in high-risk pregnancies before getting pregnant. This doctor can assess for and manage health risks during pregnancy and work with your MPN care team.

High-risk pregnancy is when you have had a blood clot, bleeding due to PV or ET, or related problems during prior pregnancies.

Pregnancy care for standard-risk disease includes:

- Taking a baby aspirin every day until the baby is born.
- After birth, receiving low-molecular-weight heparin (LMWH) for 6 weeks.
- Re-starting aspirin when LMWH is finished.

Pregnancy care for high-risk disease includes:

- After a positive pregnancy test, taking baby aspirin every day.
- Receiving LMWH throughout pregnancy and for 6 weeks after giving birth.
- If blood counts are high, lowering them with interferon or peginterferon alfa-2a.

Pregnancy care for everyone who can get pregnant includes:

- Avoiding hydroxyurea while trying to get pregnant, during pregnancy, or while breastfeeding. Hydroxyurea may harm your baby.
- Possibly taking peginterferon alfa-2a to lower blood counts, but research on its use during pregnancy is needed.

Safe anticoagulants (commonly referred to as blood thinners) that can be taken while breastfeeding are unfractionated heparin, LMWH, warfarin, and fondaparinux. Direct oral anticoagulants should be avoided.

If you have PV, the hematocrit target is based on the trimester. Hematocrit should be under 41% for the first trimester, under 38% for the second trimester, and under 39% for the third trimester.

Warning signs of blood clots

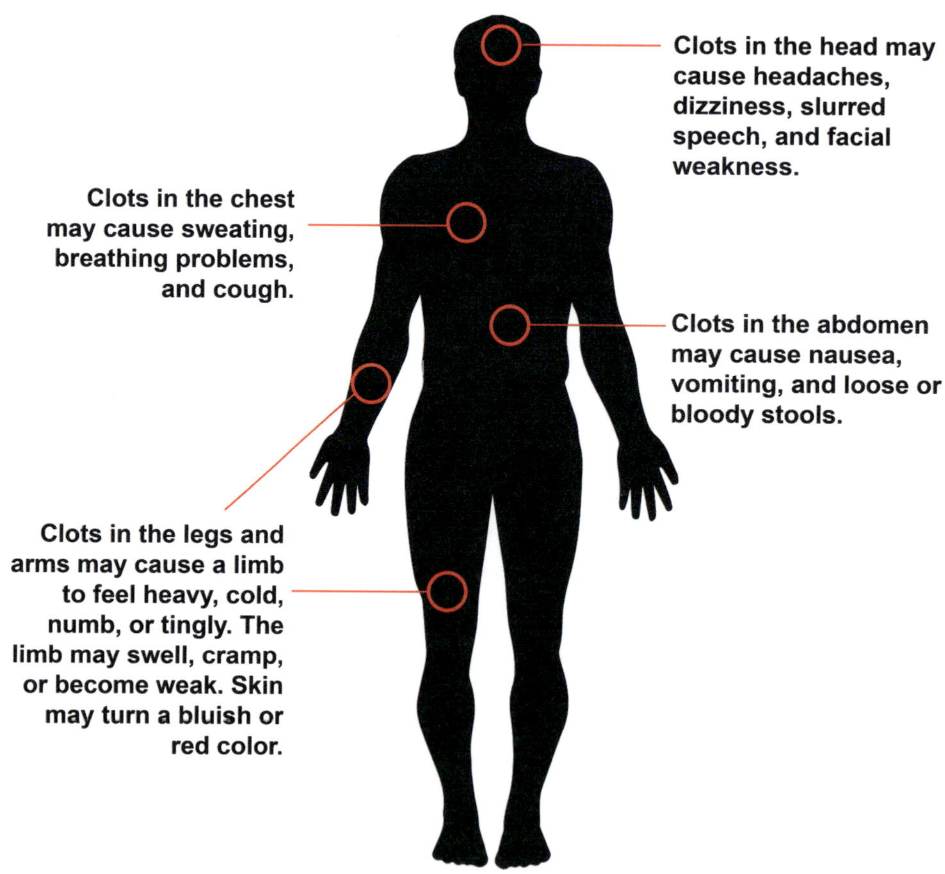

Blood clots and surgery

Surgery increases the chance for blood clots and bleeding. Your surgeon may contact your MPN team to get your health history.

Your surgeon needs to know about any blood clots, bleeding, and medications.

Before surgery, your blood counts should be close to normal to prevent blood clots and bleeding.

- You may be put on antiplatelets and cytoreductive therapy before surgery.
- People with PV may need more phlebotomies to keep your hematocrit below 45% for 3 months before surgery.
- If the surgery has a high risk for venous thromboembolism, you may be given LMWH.

Before surgery, you will need to stop taking some medicines. Aspirin is stopped 1 week before surgery.

You may stay on cytoreductive therapy until the surgery unless your surgeon tells you to stop. They will figure out when you need to stop the anticoagulant depending on how long it stays in your body.

After surgery, you will be monitored for blood clots and bleeding. You may restart your medicines if the bleeding risk is low. Aspirin is restarted 24 hours after surgery.

PV and ET checkups

After starting preventive care, you will need to meet with your care team often. Your team will assess if the MPN is causing health problems and if it's progressing. They will also assess the results of treatment.

Visits with your care team

During visits, you will be asked about new or worsening symptoms and new diagnoses. You may be given a symptom survey called the MPN-10 to complete. For information on treating symptoms, read *Chapter 6: Supportive care*.

If you have PV, your health care provider will want to know how many phlebotomies you've had since the last visit.

Your health care provider will perform a physical exam of your body. The size of your spleen and liver will be checked. Your health care provider will look for signs of blood clots and bleeding.

Blood work may be needed. Your health care provider will monitor your blood counts and other blood values. Liver and kidney function tests may be ordered as well. A peripheral blood smear may occasionally be done. Bone marrow biopsy and aspiration may be needed to rule out progression to myelofibrosis.

Changing treatments

Your treatment will likely not change if symptoms greatly improve. However, little to no relief in symptoms or worsening symptoms may trigger a treatment change. See **Guide 7** for a complete list of events that signal when a change in care may be needed.

If a change in care is needed, a clinical trial may be an option. A clinical trial is a type of medical research study. Read more about clinical trials in *Chapter 3: Types of treatment*.

If not received before, cytoreductive therapy may be the next step of care. It may be started if you now have high-risk disease, symptoms, an enlarged spleen (this is called splenomegaly and is associated with poorer health outcomes), or abnormal bleeding.

Guide 7
Events that signal that it may be time to change preventive care

Event	Polycythemia vera	Essential thrombocythemia
Blood clot	●	●
Acquired von Willebrand syndrome		●
Major bleeding	●	●
Enlarged spleen	●	●
High or increasing blood counts	●	●
New symptoms	●	●
Ongoing microvascular symptoms despite taking aspirin		●
More phlebotomies are needed to keep blood counts low, or phlebotomies are causing problems	●	
Cytoreductive therapy isn't lowering blood counts or is causing problems	●	●
Bone marrow fibrosis	●	●
Blast cells in bloodstream	●	●

Sometimes cytoreductive treatment works at first and then stops. Sometimes, it doesn't work well enough or at all. In these cases, changing to a care option listed in **Guide 8** is needed.

Guide 8
Options after initial preventive care for blood clots

	Polycythemia vera	Essential thrombocythemia
Start cytoreductive therapy if never taken before	• Clinical trial (preferred) • Ropeginterferon alfa-2b-njft (preferred) • Hydroxyurea • Peginterferon alfa-2a	• Hydroxyurea (preferred) • Peginterferon alfa-2a • Anagrelide
Stop current cytoreductive therapy and start a new treatment	• Clinical trial (preferred) • Ruxolitinib (preferred) when hydroxyurea is stopped • Ropeginterferon alfa-2b-njft, hydroxyurea, peginterferon alfa-2a if not taken before	• Clinical trial (preferred) • Hydroxyurea (preferred) if not taken before • Peginterferon alfa-2a or anagrelide if not taken before • Ruxolitinib is sometimes useful • Removing platelets from blood (plateletpheresis) in emergency situations
New treatment plan if MPN changed into myelofibrosis	Read Chapter 5 for options	Read Chapter 5 for options

Advanced/blast phase

PV and ET can progress to myelofibrosis. Progression happens in about 1 out of 10 people with PV or ET. Why these MPNs progress is unknown. Researchers are studying the role of inflammation and abnormal genes.

The risk of progression increases the longer you have PV or ET. It's rare for these MPNs to progress right into the blast phase, which is like acute myeloid leukemia (AML). If PV and ET do progress, they typically progress into chronic-phase myelofibrosis and then into advanced phases.

Once progression starts, it may be slow and take place over many years. An early sign of progression is a steady decline in the need for treatment to reduce blood counts. Your health care provider may reduce or stop treatment to see if your blood counts stop falling. If they don't, you may have myelofibrosis. Treatment of myelofibrosis is discussed in Chapter 4.

"My friend, a nurse, advised that I get a second opinion for my ET diagnosis. He went with me, and at the end he asked, 'What's the prognosis?' Doc says, 'I understand you ride a road bike and stay in shape. More than likely, if you follow your hematologist advice, you'll live 20 years, unless you get hit by a bus.' That was 12 years ago, and I am still pedaling. I am almost 79 years old."

Key points

- People with polycythemia vera (PV) and essential thrombocythemia (ET) are prone to blood clots. With preventive care, most people live for many years.
- Preventive care is based on your risk of blood clots. Having a healthy heart and blood vessels is a goal for everyone. Aspirin is also commonly used to prevent clots.
- For PV, phlebotomy is performed to reduce hematocrit. For high-risk PV/ET, cytoreductive treatment may be an option to reduce blood counts.
- Your care may change if you become pregnant and change again after giving birth.
- Your care may be changed temporarily if you need surgery because it increases the risk of clots and bleeding.
- You will need to meet with your care team often. During visits, the status of the cancer and the results of preventive care will be checked.
- If PV or ET is getting worse, your treatment may be changed. The next treatment will depend on the current clot risk level, your prior treatment, and if there is progression to myelofibrosis.

Questions to ask

- What type of MPN do I have?
- Is this a fast- or slow-growing MPN?
- What are the possible complications of MPN?

"I'm happy I found the right hematologist after 2 tries. Make sure your doctor is an MPN researcher and does the right genetic tests for mutations."

6 Supportive care

The goal of supportive care is to maintain or improve your quality of life. This chapter discusses some of the supportive needs of people with myeloproliferative neoplasms (MPNs).

Supportive care is an important part of cancer care. The goal is to improve your quality of life. Supportive care is for everyone with cancer and their loved ones, not just for those at the end of life. It's also known as palliative care.

Supportive care includes a wide range of services. Supportive care prevents or manages the symptoms of cancer and the side effects of cancer treatment, like pain and cancer-related fatigue. It also addresses the mental, social, emotional, and spiritual concerns faced by people with cancer.

Supportive care provides help with additional needs, such as:

- Making treatment decisions
- Coordinating your care
- Paying for care
- Planning for advance care and end of life

Read more about the types of support you may receive in *NCCN Guidelines for Patients: Palliative Care*, available at NCCN.org/patientguidelines and on the NCCN Patient Guides for Cancer app.

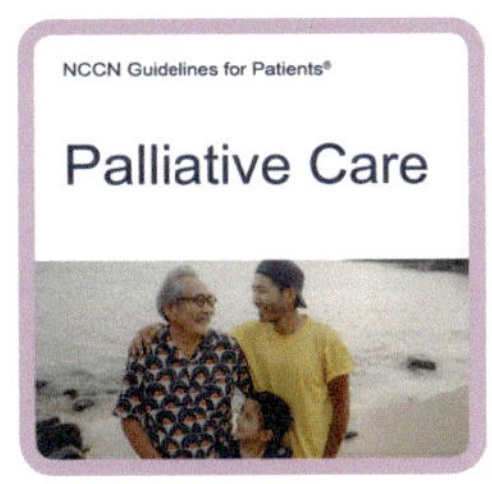

"Please ensure that your hematologist/MPN specialist listens and actually hears what you're saying. It doesn't matter what the symptoms are. You could be the first to experience something 'outside of the radar.' They're there for you."

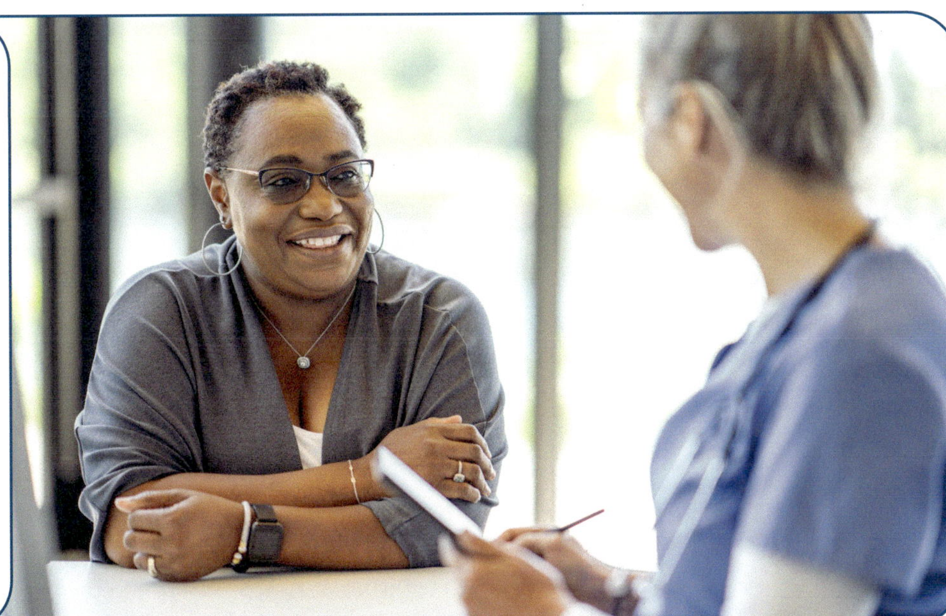

Supportive care guidelines

Distress

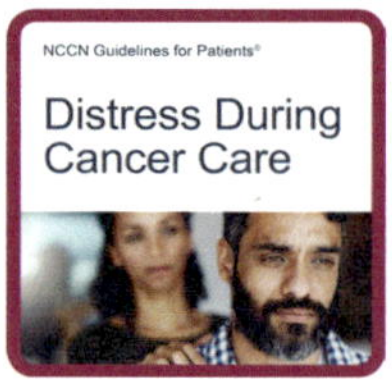

Everyone with cancer feels distress at some point. It's normal to be worried, sad, helpless, or angry. Distress can become severe and affect the way you live.

Fatigue

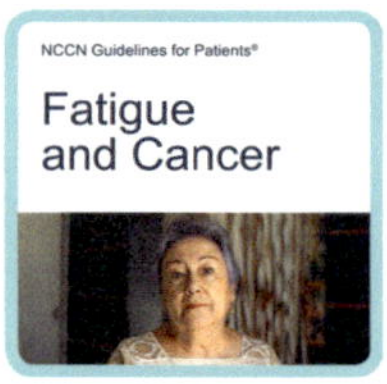

Cancer-related fatigue is not the typical tiredness that follows an active or long day—it's a lack of energy that is distressing, does not improve with normal resting or sleep, and disrupts life.

Palliative care

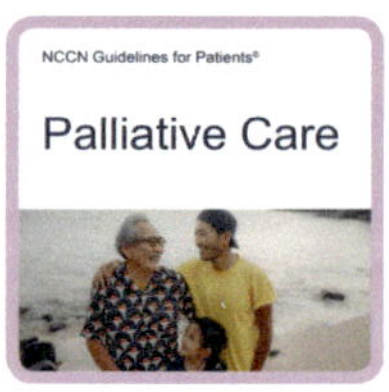

Palliative care is an approach to health care for people living with serious illnesses, including cancer. It focuses on providing relief from the symptoms and stress of having cancer.

Nausea and vomiting

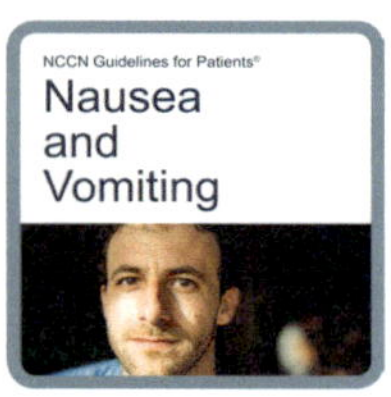

Chemotherapy can cause nausea and vomiting. Nausea is the feeling that you are going to throw up. Vomiting is forcefully throwing up what's in your stomach.

Graft-Versus-Host Disease

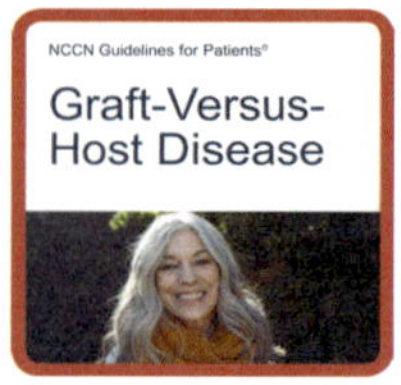

A side effect of allogeneic hematopoietic cell transplants is graft-versus-host disease. This side effect is caused by donor cells attacking your healthy cells.

Late and long-term effects

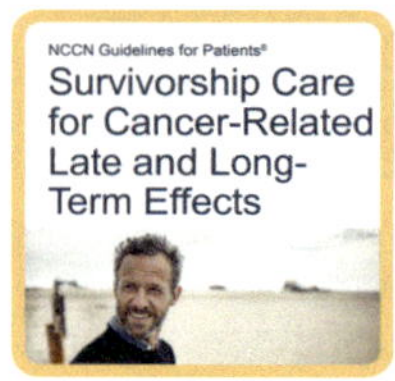

Cancer and its treatment can cause long-term and late effects. Long-term effects start during treatment and persist after treatment is done. Late effects are less common and start long after treatment has ended. Long-term and late effects include heart disease, fatigue, poor sleep, pain, and depression.

Healthy living

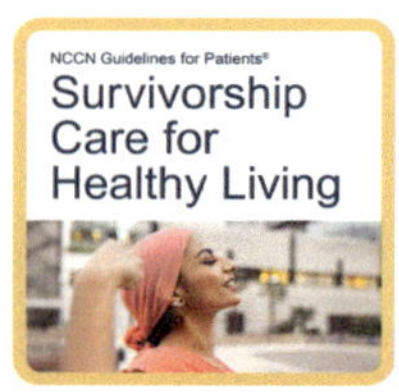

It's important to start or keep a healthy lifestyle. Healthy living may help prevent disease and improve well-being. This guide discusses physical activity, food, and vaccinations.

The full library of NCCN Guidelines for Patients is available at NCCN.org/patientguidelines

Bleeding

People with myeloproliferative neoplasms (MPNs) are at increased risk of bleeding, also called hemorrhaging. However, bleeding is often mild. Bleeding in patients with MPNs can be confusing even to physicians because your platelet counts could be high or low. Sometimes even when your bone marrow produces an excess of platelets, they do not work as well as normal to clot the blood.

Bleeding occurs more often in myelofibrosis than in polycythemia vera (PV) and essential thrombocythemia (ET). It can be severe, especially in people who have anemia or low platelet counts.

Bleeding events differ among people. Some people bruise easily, while others get nose bleeds. Menstrual periods may be heavier than normal. You may have bleeding in your digestive tract. You may see blood in your urine.

Ask your care team which types of bleeding events need immediate medical attention.

Causes of bleeding

Normally, bleeding is stopped when cells called platelets plug the hole in blood vessels with help from clotting factors. A lot of bleeding may occur when the blood doesn't clot properly.

There are several causes of bleeding in PV and ET:

- Platelets may not work correctly.
- The number of platelets may be very high. High levels of platelets may lower a clotting factor called von Willebrand.
- Prevention of blood clots with aspirin may thin the blood too much.
- Prevention of blood clots with antiplatelet or cytoreductive therapy may reduce blood counts to very low levels.
- Treating blood clots with anticoagulants may slow down clotting time too much.

The cause of bleeding is simpler in myelofibrosis—bleeding is typically caused by a low number of platelets.

Bleeding in myelofibrosis

You may receive a platelet transfusion to prevent bleeding if your platelet count is lower than 10,000 m3. Platelet transfusions are also used to treat bleeding. Most white blood cells are removed during the donation process. This helps prevent the blood from attacking your body. It also prevents infection with cytomegalovirus (CMV).

Transfusions may not stop bleeding. In this case, antifibrinolytic agents may be used. These drugs help your blood to clot.

Bleeding in PV and ET

Your health care provider will identify and treat all causes of bleeding. Coagulation tests to assess for acquired von Willebrand syndrome may be done. Levels of von Willebrand factor may be low due to high platelet counts.

Aspirin will be stopped until the platelet count is normal. Treatment to reduce platelet counts may be given. If you have ET, you may receive plateletpheresis if bleeding is severe, but this is rare.

Blood clots

You may get a blood clot even though you took steps to prevent it. Many blood clots are safely managed with anticoagulants. Coagulation is another word for blood clotting. Despite being called blood thinners, anticoagulants slow down the clotting of blood.

Anticoagulants

Research has shown that anticoagulants help treat blood clots in general practice. But there is little to no research on anticoagulants in people with an MPN. It's unknown if one anticoagulant works better than another. It's also unknown exactly how long an anticoagulant is needed.

Your health care provider will decide how long you'll take an anticoagulant based on the severity of the blood clot. Three common types of anticoagulant are:

- **Low-molecular-weight heparin (LMWH)** – This medicine enhances the effect of a natural anticoagulant in your body. It's injected into the skin, which can be done at home.
- **Direct oral anticoagulants** – These pills disable proteins that help the blood to clot. They include apixaban (Eliquis), betrixaban (Bevyxxa), dabigatran (Pradaxa), edoxaban (Savaysa), and rivaroxaban (Xarelto).
- **Vitamin K blockers** – Among these medicines, warfarin (Coumadin, Jantoven) is the most often used. It's a pill taken at home. Warfarin stops the liver from using vitamin K, which is needed to make clotting proteins. When you are taking warfarin, regular testing will be necessary to measure how quickly or slowly your blood is clotting.

Anticoagulants increase the risk of bleeding. The risk is higher if you are taking aspirin or having treatment that lowers platelet counts. Your health care provider may stop these treatments while you're on an anticoagulant. People with cardiovascular risk factors may stay on aspirin, but this may change depending on the situation.

Plateletpheresis

If you have a sudden life-threatening clot, you may receive plateletpheresis. This procedure withdraws your blood and removes platelets. Your platelet-reduced blood will then be returned to your body.

Plateletpheresis is rarely done because it only slightly decreases platelets and for a short time. It's useful in ET when people have life-threatening bleeds or clots or are not responding to medication.

> **“Knowledge is power. Do not settle if your questions and concerns are not properly addressed. There are many skilled MPN specialists throughout the nation that can provide relief, comfort, and improved quality of life. Advocate for yourself and your needs."**

Bone pain

Your health care provider will evaluate if any bone pain is caused by the MPN. This is needed because treatment of MPN-related bone pain differs from treatment of joint pain.

In one MPN study, ruxolitinib stabilized bone and muscle pain. For some people, loratadine and non-steroidal anti-inflammatory drugs (NSAIDs) may provide relief. A low dose of radiation may provide short-term relief of bone pain.

Headaches and tinnitus

Starting to have headaches may mean you have a blood clot. A high-pitched ringing in your ears not heard by others may also be a symptom of a blood clot. Tell your health care provider if you have these symptoms.

Headaches as well as other vascular symptoms may be relieved with low-dose aspirin. If symptoms persist, taking aspirin twice a day or taking an antiplatelet agent (clopidogrel) may have better results. Aspirin may be given with an antiplatelet agent. Taking an NSAID with aspirin should be done with caution and not without your physician's knowledge. Always tell an urgent care or emergency care practitioner if you are taking daily aspirin.

There are several options in addition to aspirin. Headaches in people with PV may be relieved with phlebotomy or ruxolitinib. For all MPNs, cytoreduction therapy reduces headaches and other vascular symptoms. Migraine headaches may be treated and possibly prevented with triptans or topiramate.

Itching

Itching (pruritus) is a common problem among people with MPNs. It can be severe, even life altering.

The first approach to relieve itching is to practice care for sensitive skin. This includes taking short showers, using mild soap, and moisturizing your skin. Antihistamines (cetirizine, diphenhydramine) and topical steroids may also be helpful.

If needed, the next step to relieve itching will be based on the benefits and downsides of treatments. Ruxolitinib relieves itching. Early research on selective serotonin reuptake inhibitors (SSRIs) and narrow-band ultraviolet B shows promise.

Other medicines that may be tried include peginterferon alfa-2a; gabapentin; aprepitant; and immunosuppressant agents, such as cyclosporine, methotrexate, azathioprine, mycophenolate mofetil, or dupilumab.

Infections

You may be prone to infections because of myelofibrosis or its treatment. Ask your health care provider which vaccinations are safe for you. If you're taking a JAK inhibitor, they may prescribe the recombinant (killed) zoster vaccine, more commonly known as the shingles vaccine.

If you get infections often, your health care provider may prescribe antibiotics for prevention. If you have low neutrophil counts, instead of antibiotics you may receive granulocyte colony-stimulating factor (G-CSF) or granulocyte-macrophage colony-stimulating factor (GM-CSF).

Tumor lysis syndrome

Tumor lysis syndrome (TLS) occurs when the waste released by dead cells is not quickly cleared out of the body. The waste can cause kidney damage and severe blood electrolyte disturbances. TLS can be life-threatening.

Induction chemotherapy may cause TLS. This type of chemotherapy is a treatment for advanced myelofibrosis or acute myeloid leukemia (AML). This treatment kills many cancer cells and results in too much waste too quickly.

TLS may be prevented by high amounts of fluids during chemotherapy. Fluids may help clear out the cell waste. Decreasing uric acid levels with allopurinol or rasburicase is another option. Rasburicase may be given as the first treatment if you have high uric acid or if it's affecting your kidneys.

Iron overload

Iron overload means there's too much iron in your body. It can occur if you've had many red blood cell transfusions. Iron chelation is a type of drug that removes extra iron from your body. It's an option at times for lower-risk myelofibrosis. Your health care provider may prescribe iron chelation if you've had more than 20 transfusions since diagnosis or your blood ferritin level is greater than 2500 ng/mL.

Supportive care guidelines

The library of NCCN Guidelines for Patients has several guides on supportive care. These guides focus on the treatment of common physical and emotional effects of many cancers. One guide is about healthy living and shares recommendations for exercise, food and supplements, and vaccines.

“ I am now in my 10th year after a diagnosis of PV and only within the last month or so changed my daily regime of hydroxyurea 500 mg two times a day. I am fortunate in being largely asymptomatic, though the hydroxyurea does cause skin issues! Learn all you can about MPNs, be persistent in your questions, and be comfortable with your oncologist."

Key points

- Supportive care is health care that improves quality of life. It provides symptom relief and help for other needs, such as stress reduction, mental health support, and financial and health insurance assistance.
- Bleeding is more common in myelofibrosis than in polycythemia vera (PV) and essential thrombocytopenia (ET). Treatment options vary among myeloproliferative neoplasm (MPN) types to target the cause of bleeding.
- Blood clots are a focus of prevention and treatment for PV and ET, but blood clots also occur in people with myelofibrosis. They are treated with anticoagulants and antiplatelet medicines.
- Bone pain, headaches, tinnitus, and itching occur across all MPNs and can greatly impact quality of life. Approved medications and drugs in clinical trials can help with these symptoms. Significant research is underway to find the best treatment for individuals with these MPN-related symptoms.
- People with myelofibrosis may develop frequent infections, tumor lysis syndrome, and high levels of iron. Vaccinations may be your best defense against infections. Fluids to clear out cell waste may prevent tumor lysis syndrome (TLS). Iron chelation is a treatment for high levels of iron.

Questions to ask

- What are the possible complications and side effects of treatment?
- Which side effects are most common and how long do they usually last?
- Which side effects are serious or life-threatening?
- Are there any long-term or permanent side effects?

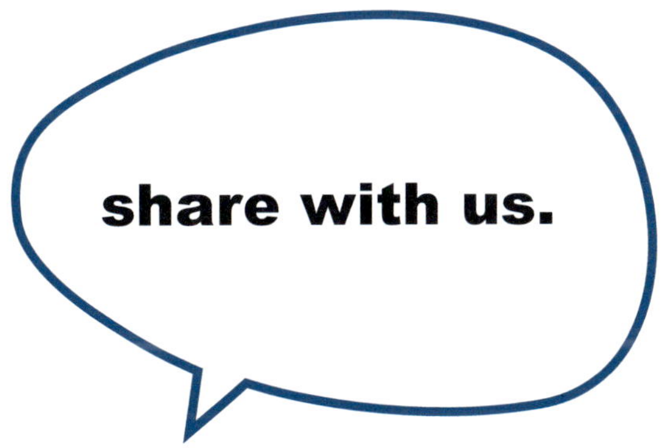

Take our survey and help make the NCCN Guidelines for Patients better for everyone!

NCCN.org/patients/comments

7 Other resources

Want to learn more? Here's how you can get additional help.

What else to know

This guide helps you know your options so you can make informed decisions and improve your cancer care. But it's not the only resource that you have.

Ask for as much information and help as you need. Many people are interested in learning more about:

- The details of myeloproliferative neoplasm (MPN) treatments and their side effects
- Being a part of a care team
- Getting financial help
- Finding a cancer care professional who's an expert in their field
- Coping with other health problems

What else to do

Your health care center can help you with next steps. It often has on-site resources to help meet your needs and find answers to your questions. Health care centers can also inform you of resources in your community.

In addition to help from your providers, the resources listed in the next section provide support for many people like yourself.

Where to get help

Look through the list below and visit the provided websites to learn more about these organizations.

AnCan Foundation
ancan.org

Blood Cancer United
bloodcancerunited.org

Cancer*Care*
cancercare.org

HealthTree Foundation
healthtree.org

Imerman Angels
imermanangels.org

***MPN* Cancer Connection**
mpncancerconnection.org

MPN Research Foundation
mpnresearchfoundation.org

NMDP
nmdp.org

TargetCancer Foundation
targetcancer.org

Triage Cancer
triagecancer.org

Questions to ask

- Who can I talk to about help with stress/mental health, housing, food, and other basic needs?
- What assistance is available for transportation, childcare, and home care?
- Who can tell me what my options for health insurance are and assist me with applying for insurance coverage?
- How much will I have to pay for my treatment? What help is available to pay for medicines and other treatment?
- Who can help me with my concerns about work or school?

"The initial diagnosis and new reality can be very overwhelming since not much is known about MPNs. While myelofibrosis is very rare, there are helpful resources from MPN research and education organizations as well as informal patient networks that provide the opportunity to share questions, fears, symptoms, and treatments. It is comforting to know there is new research and potential treatment options emerging that should help improve and extend our lives."

Words to know

acute myeloid leukemia (AML)
Blood cancer of young white blood cells called myeloblasts, or blasts.

allogeneic hematopoietic cell transplant (HCT)
Cancer treatment that replaces blood stem cells with donor stem cells, which in turn make new, healthy bone marrow.

anemia
Low levels of healthy red blood cells that cannot provide enough oxygen to tissue.

anticoagulant
A treatment that slows the clotting of blood.

BCR-ABL1
An abnormal gene that is the hallmark of chronic myeloid leukemia.

biomarker test
A lab test of a molecule in your body to assess your health.

blast
An early form of a blood cell that is unable to function like a mature blood cell, also called myeloblasts.

blood clot
A gel-like clump of blood. Also called a thrombus.

blood smear
A test that involves viewing a drop of blood with a microscope to assess features of blood cells.

bone marrow
A soft, spongy material inside of bones where most blood cells are made.

bone marrow aspiration
Removal of a small amount of liquid bone marrow to test for disease.

bone marrow biopsy
Removal of a small amount of solid bone and bone marrow to test for disease.

chromosome
A long, tightly coiled structure in cells that contains coded instructions for cell behavior.

chronic myeloid leukemia (CML)
Blood cancer that causes too many white blood cells called granulocytes to form.

clinical trial
Research on a test or treatment to assess its safety or how well it works.

coagulation test
A test of the proteins that cause blood to clot.

complete blood count (CBC)
A test of the number of blood cells in a sample.

comprehensive metabolic panel
Tests of up to 14 chemicals in your blood.

constitutional symptom
A physical condition that is a general effect of a disease.

cytogenetics
The study of chromosomes using a microscope.

cytomegalovirus (CMV)
A virus that can be transmitted through donated white blood cells.

cytoreductive therapy
A treatment that reduces the number of blood cells.

diabetes
A disease that causes high levels of blood sugar.

diagnosis
Identification of an illness based on tests.

differential
Measurement of the different types of white blood cells in a blood sample.

Dynamic International Prognostic Scoring System (DIPSS)
A scoring system for the prognosis of people with primary myelofibrosis.

embolus
A blood clot that is not attached to a base and moves through the bloodstream.

erythropoiesis-stimulating agent
A drug that helps bone marrow to make more red blood cells.

erythropoietin (EPO)
A hormone made by the kidneys.

essential thrombocythemia (ET)
A type of cancer in which blood stem cells make too many platelets. Also called essential thrombocytosis.

fatigue
A feeling of extreme tiredness, even with enough sleep, that limits a person's ability to function.

fibrosis
Scarring of supportive fibers in tissue.

fluorescence in situ hybridization (FISH)
A lab test that uses special dyes to look for abnormal changes in a cell's genes and chromosomes.

gene
A set of coded instructions in cells that controls cell behavior.

graft-versus-host disease (GVHD)
An attack on normal cells by blood stem cells from a donor.

granulocyte
A type of white blood cell.

granulocyte colony-stimulating factor (G-CSF)/granulocyte-macrophage colony-stimulating factor (GM-CSF)
Medicines given to people who get infections often and have low neutrophil counts.

hematocrit
The percentage of red cells in blood.

hematopathologist
A health care provider who's an expert at diagnosing cancers of the blood and immune system.

hematopoietic cell
A cell from which all other types of blood cells are made. Also called blood stem cell.

hemoglobin
A protein in red blood cells that carries oxygen.

hemorrhage
Blood loss inside or outside of the body. Also called bleeding.

human leukocyte antigen (HLA)
Special proteins on the surface of cells that help the body to tell its own cells apart from foreign cells.

hypertension
High blood pressure.

International Prognostic Score of Thrombosis (IPSET)
A risk stratification tool for people with essential thrombocytopenia.

iron
A mineral needed to make new red blood cells.

karyotype
A test that uses a microscope to examine a cell's chromosomes.

lactate dehydrogenase (LDH)
A protein that helps to make energy in cells.

leukocyte
A type of white blood cell.

liver function tests
Tests that measure chemicals made or processed by the liver.

low-molecular-weight heparin (LMWH)
A medicine given to prevent blood clots.

medical history
A report of all your health events and medications.

megakaryocyte
A bone marrow cell that makes platelets.

molecular test
A lab test of an abnormal gene inside of cells.

mutation
An abnormal set of coded instructions in a gene.

Mutation-Enhanced International Prognostic Score System (MIPSS)
A system used to estimate risk of disease progression and/or complications in people with primary myelofibrosis.

myeloproliferative neoplasm (MPN)
A cancer of blood-forming cells that causes an excess of blood cells or bone marrow scarring.

myelofibrosis
Scarring of the bone marrow not due to other bone marrow problems.

Myelofibrosis Secondary to PV and ET-Prognostic Model (MYSEC-PM)
A risk stratification system used for post-polycythemia vera and post-essential thrombocythemia myelofibrosis.

paresthesia
A burning or prickling sensation in the body.

pathologist
A doctor who's an expert in testing cells and tissue to find disease.

phlebotomy
Withdrawal of blood.

physical exam
A review of the body by a health expert for signs of disease.

platelet
A type of blood cell that helps control bleeding. Also called thrombocyte.

plateletpheresis
A procedure that withdraws blood, removes platelets, and then returns your altered blood to your body.

polycythemia vera (PV)
Cancer of blood-forming cells that causes too many red blood cells.

post-ET myelofibrosis
Advanced essential thrombocythemia with scarring in the bone marrow.

post-PV myelofibrosis
Advanced polycythemia vera with scarring in the bone marrow.

primary myelofibrosis (PMF)
A person's first MPN, which is also not caused by PV or ET.

prognosis
The likely course and outcome of a disease based on tests.

progression
Worsening of cancer.

pruritus
Itchy skin.

reverse transcription-polymerase chain reaction (RT-PCR)
A lab test that detects a cancer marker even if it's in only a few cells.

risk stratification
An assessment of the likelihood of an event based on proven predictors.

spleen
A small organ to the left of your stomach that is part of the immune system.

splenomegaly
An abnormally large spleen.

supportive care
Treatment for the symptoms or health conditions caused by cancer or cancer treatment.

thrombosis
Clots that can block blood flow in blood vessels.

tinnitus
A high-pitched ringing in your ears not heard by others.

tumor lysis syndrome (TLS)
A health condition caused by rapid death of many cancer cells.

uric acid
A chemical that is in most cells.

vein
A blood vessel that moves blood back to the heart.

venous thromboembolism
A blood clot that forms in a deep vein that may now be stuck in a lung artery.

von Willebrand syndrome (VWS)
A blood disorder that causes blood not to clot.

We want your feedback!

Our goal is to provide helpful and easy-to-understand information on cancer.
Take our survey to let us know what we got right and what we could do better.
NCCN.org/patients/feedback

NCCN Contributors

This patient guide is based on the NCCN Clinical Practice Guidelines in Oncology (NCCN Guidelines®) for Myeloproliferative Neoplasms, Version 1.2026. It was adapted, reviewed, and published with help from the following people:

Dorothy A. Shead, MS
Senior Director
Patient Information Operations

Tim Rinehart
Medical Writer

Lisa Diehl
Production Layout Artist

The NCCN Clinical Practice Guidelines in Oncology (NCCN Guidelines®) for Myeloproliferative Neoplasms, Version 1.2026, were developed by the following NCCN Panel Members:

T. Gerds, MD, MS/Chair
Case Comprehensive Cancer Center/ UniversityHospitals Seidman Cancer Center and Cleveland Clinic Taussig Cancer Institute

Jason Gotlib, MD, MS/Vice-Chair
Stanford Cancer Institute

Peter Abdelmessieh, DO, MSc
Fox Chase Cancer Center

*Haris Ali, MD
City of Hope National Medical Center

Mariana Castells, MD, PhD
Dana-Farber/Brigham and Women's Cancer Center

Brian J. Chernak, MD
Memorial Sloan Kettering Cancer Center

Manuel R. Espinoza-Gutarra, MD
O'Neal Comprehensive Cancer Center at UAB

*Ruth Fein Revell, BS
Patient advocate

Steven Green, MD
Roswell Park Comprehensive Cancer Center

Krishna Gundabolu, MBBS, MS
Fred & Pamela Buffett Cancer Center

Elizabeth Hexner, MD, MS
Abramson Cancer Center at the University of Pennsylvania

Tania Jain, MBBS
Johns Hopkins Kimmel Cancer Center

Catriona H. Jamieson, MD, PhD
UC San Diego Moores Cancer Center

Irum Khan, MD
Robert H. Lurie Comprehensive Cancer Center of Northwestern University

Andrew T. Kuykendall, MD
Moffitt Cancer Center

Yazan F. Madanat, MD
UT Southwestern Simmons Comprehensive Cancer Center

Lucia Masarova, MD
The University of Texas MD Anderson Cancer Center

Brandon McMahon, MD
University of Colorado Cancer Center

Sanjay R. Mohan, MD, MSCI
Vanderbilt-Ingram Cancer Center

Kalyan V. Nadiminti, MD
University of Wisconsin Carbone Cancer Center

Stephen Oh, MD, PhD
Siteman Cancer Center at Barnes-Jewish Hospital and Washington University School of Medicine

Jeanne Palmer
Mayo Clinic Comprehensive Cancer Center

Ami B. Patel, MD
Huntsman Cancer Institute at the University of Utah

*Anand A. Patel, MD
The UChicago Medicine Comprehensive Cancer Center

Nikolai Podoltsev, MD, PhD
Yale Cancer Center/Smilow Cancer Hospital

Lindsay Rein, MD
Duke Cancer Institute

Rachel Salit, MD
Fred Hutchinson Cancer Center

Mary Sehl, MD
UCLA Jonsson Comprehensive Cancer Center

Moshe Talpaz, MD
University of Michigan Rogel Cancer Center

Martha Wadleigh, MD
Dana-Farber/Brigham and Women's Cancer Center

Sarah A. Wall, MD, MPH
The Ohio State University Comprehensive Cancer Center - James Cancer Hospital and Solove Research Institute

NCCN

Mary Anne Bergman
Guidelines Coordinator

Cindy Hochstetler, PhD
Oncology Scientist/Senior Medical Writer

* Reviewed this patient guide. For disclosures, visit NCCN.org/disclosures.

NCCN Cancer Centers

For contact information, visit NCCN.org/cancercenters.

Abramson Cancer Center
at the University of Pennsylvania
Philadelphia, Pennsylvania

Case Comprehensive Cancer Center/
University Hospitals Seidman Cancer Center and
Cleveland Clinic Taussig Cancer Institute
Cleveland, Ohio

City of Hope National Medical Center
Duarte, California

Dana-Farber/Brigham and Women's Cancer Center |
Mass General Cancer Center
Boston, Massachusetts

Duke Cancer Institute
Durham, North Carolina

Fox Chase Cancer Center
Philadelphia, Pennsylvania

Fred & Pamela Buffett Cancer Center
Omaha, Nebraska

Fred Hutchinson Cancer Center
Seattle, Washington

Huntsman Cancer Institute at the University of Utah
Salt Lake City, Utah

Indiana University Melvin and Bren Simon
Comprehensive Cancer Center
Indianapolis, Indiana

Johns Hopkins Kimmel Cancer Center
Baltimore, Maryland

Mayo Clinic Comprehensive Cancer Center
Phoenix/Scottsdale, Arizona
Jacksonville, Florida
Rochester, Minnesota

Memorial Sloan Kettering Cancer Center
New York, New York

Moffitt Cancer Center
Tampa, Florida

O'Neal Comprehensive Cancer Center at UAB
Birmingham, Alabama

Robert H. Lurie Comprehensive Cancer Center
of Northwestern University
Chicago, Illinois

Roswell Park Comprehensive Cancer Center
Buffalo, New York

Siteman Cancer Center at Barnes-Jewish Hospital
and Washington University School of Medicine
St. Louis, Missouri

St. Jude Children's Research Hospital/
The University of Tennessee Health Science Center
Memphis, Tennessee

Stanford Cancer Institute
Stanford, California

The Ohio State University Comprehensive Cancer Center -
James Cancer Hospital and Solove Research Institute
Columbus, Ohio

The UChicago Medicine Comprehensive Cancer Center
Chicago, Illinois

The University of Texas MD Anderson Cancer Center
Houston, Texas

UC Davis Comprehensive Cancer Center
Sacramento, California

UC San Diego Moores Cancer Center
La Jolla, California

UCLA Jonsson Comprehensive Cancer Center
Los Angeles, California

UCSF Helen Diller Family Comprehensive Cancer Center
San Francisco, California

University of Colorado Cancer Center
Aurora, Colorado

University of Michigan Rogel Cancer Center
Ann Arbor, Michigan

University of Wisconsin Carbone Cancer Center
Madison, Wisconsin

UT Southwestern Simmons
Comprehensive Cancer Center
Dallas, Texas

Vanderbilt-Ingram Cancer Center
Nashville, Tennessee

Yale Cancer Center/Smilow Cancer Hospital
New Haven, Connecticut

Index

Let us know what you think!

Please take a moment to complete an online survey about the NCCN Guidelines for Patients.
NCCN.org/patients/response

Made in the USA
Monee, IL
14 September 2026

62771515R00040